Cytomegalovirus

Cunningham’s

HERVÉ GUIBERT

Cytomegalovirus

A Hospitalization Diary

Introduction by
David Caron

Afterword by
Todd Meyers

Translated by
Clara Orban

Fordham University Press
New York   2016

Forms of Living | Stefanos Geroulanos and Todd Meyers, series editors

Copyright © 1996 by University Press of America, Inc.

First Fordham University Press edition, 2016

Fordham University Press has no responsibility for the persistence or accuracy of
URLs for external or third-party Internet websites referred to in this publication and
does not guarantee that any content on such websites is, or will remain, accurate or
appropriate.

Fordham University Press also publishes its books in a variety of electronic formats.
Some content that appears in print may not be available in electronic books.

Visit us online at www.fordhampress.com.

Library of Congress Cataloging-in-Publication Data
  Guibert, Hervé.
  [Cytomegalovirus. English]
  Cytomegalovirus : a hospitalization diary / Hervé Guibert, Todd Meyers ;
introduction by David Caron ; translated by Clara Orban ; introduction by David
Caron ; afterword by Todd Meyers.—First Fordham University Press edition.
      pages cm.—(Forms of living)
  Includes bibliographical references.
  ISBN 978-0-8232-6856-6 (hardback) — ISBN 978-0-8232-6857-3 (paper)
    1. AIDS (Disease)—Patients—Biography. 2. Cytomegalovirus infections—
Patients—France—Diaries. 3. Hospital patients—France—Diaries. 4. Authors—
France—Diaries. 5. Eye—Infections—Patients—France—Diaries. 6. AIDS
(Disease)—Complications—Patients—France—Diaries. I. Title.
  RC136.8.G8513 2016
  362.19697'920092—dc23
  [B]

                                   2015017379

Printed in the United States of America

18 17 16   5 4 3 2 1

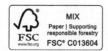

CONTENTS

Introduction: Respect, One Dessert Spoon at a Time   1
David Caron

CYTOMEGALOVIRUS: A Hospitalization Diary   27

Afterword: Remainders   75
Todd Meyers

Translator's Note   83

Cytomegalovirus

Respect, One Dessert Spoon at a Time

DAVID CARON

There is an extraordinary scene in Hervé Guibert's short, unsparing hospital diary, *Cytomegalovirus*. Hervé, the narrator, is being prepped for the eye operation that could add some time and a degree of comfort to his life but might also make him—a photographer and lover of beautiful boys—lose his sight. "There is an eye at stake," he notes, and it sounds almost like an understatement. Cytomegalovirus, a form of herpes normally harmless to otherwise healthy people, killed a great number of people with AIDS at the time the book takes place. And Hervé is so ill, so weak. In fact, as he is writing these lines, the young author has about two months to live. But when a nurse he loathes barges into his hospital room before the operation to demand that he put on a transparent paper gown with nothing underneath, except maybe his briefs if he insists, he flat-out refuses: "You'll have to wait until I'm a lot worse off than I am now to get me to walk through a hospital in this thing." After a brief confrontation, he walks down the hallways to the operating room in his street clothes, hat and all. Of course, when he gets there the orderlies have no idea who he is. How could they? They expected a patient and they had to acknowledge a person. Eventually, Hervé changes into the same outfit they are wearing. The clothes make the man, it seems, in more ways than one.

This brief passage in this tiny book has always had a tremendous effect on me, as strong perhaps as the two earlier masterpieces that made Hervé Guibert a literary sensation literally overnight, after he appeared on a television literary talk show: *To the Friend Who Did Not Save My Life* and *The Compassion Protocol*. In many ways, Guibert, who already had a dozen other books behind him but few readers, gave AIDS a public face at a time when the epidemic was raging with no relief in sight. It was 1990. By the end of 1991, he was dead at the age of thirty-six. To this day, Guibert's remains one of the most important artistic voices to come out of the AIDS epidemic in France and, arguably, beyond, while posthumous publications of his work keep meeting enthusiastic critical and commercial reception. And to this day, I keep returning for inspiration to the slim volume that was released in 1992, shortly after his death.

I'm quite serious about this: I had brain surgery not long

ago, and when the nurses told me I had to be naked under the gown before going to the operating room, I instantly channeled Guibert. I demanded to know why on earth I needed to be bare-assed for a procedure that would take place through my nose. Then they explained all the other stuff that comes with an operation like that and it all made sense, so OK, fine, I'll get naked. I didn't actually mind, to be honest with you, but I resisted, and that's what counts.

In the two-week diary of the hospital stay that makes up *Cytomegalovirus*, Hervé can sometimes come across as a difficult patient, the kind who nags nurses and complains endlessly about the most mundane problems. Mundane to most of us, of course, but when you are so weak that the slightest infection can kill you, you live in a world where nothing is ever mundane. The crummy IV pole with a broken wheel doesn't move as it should and thus restricts Hervé's movements and freedom. His room hasn't been cleaned properly before his arrival, and there's even dirty stuff under the bed. One evening, he is given a single spoon with which to eat both his soup and his dessert. And so on. . . . That last bit often fails to provoke my students' compassion ("Il est très . . . Comment dit-on *petty?*"), until I explain that, in French cuisine, you don't normally mix sweet and savory, and it isn't customary to use the same utensils for both. Expecting Hervé to do so—worse even, not even entertaining the thought that he could mind, just as the hospital employees themselves mind once they're eating at home and out of their work uniforms—constitutes therefore a symbolic form of social exclusion as brutal to him as it is innocuous-looking to his indifferent nurses. What somebody on one side endows with tremendous value appears all but worthless on the other, where people use spoons to eat, not symbolize. A missing utensil may not seem as offensive to human dignity as forced public nakedness, but for Hervé the two pertain to the same system and serve the same immediate goal: the organized humiliation and subjugation of patients within an institution whose purpose, it seems, is to do just that.

Hervé doesn't explicitly connect his litany of complaints to his particular status as a gay man living with AIDS. "Hospitals are hell," he remarks as he describes the constant noise and movement that make hospital nights indistinguishable from hospital days. It is true that homosexual men have had a fraught relation with doctors from the moment modern science invented both, and it is also true that AIDS brought that century-old face-off to a previously unseen level of tension and ambiguity. How safe are you supposed to feel when you have to place your life in the hands of the very people you have learned to identify as a principal enemy? Still, numerous other patients could have made a similar observation about hospitals, whatever health issue sent them to one. Guibert critiques the hospital as an institution of power and a battleground for supremacy: "You have to make them respect you right away, it's exhausting, a test of wills that lasts one or even several days and nights. They want you to lose, they count on wearing you down. Then, according to the situation, they respect or they flatten you." And to remove any doubts as to its author's intentions, the diary includes passing mentions of Guibert's friend Michel Foucault, referred to as "M" in the text but whose identity has become transparent to readers since Guibert told of Foucault's death from AIDS in *To the Friend Who Did Not Save My Life.* Hervé, in other words, is not a naïve patient, and his defiance conveys more than just annoyance.

In a sense, that Guibert's account of his hospital stay should focus so little on AIDS per se may explain why the book's appeal has endured, perhaps even broadened. Not that it somehow transcends AIDS or universalizes the experience of it, but the political fight for dignity against institutional indifference needs to be waged on many fronts at once. Still, Guibert did have AIDS, he wrote about AIDS, he died of AIDS. Some French activists criticized him for what they saw as apolitical and romantic self-involvement, but by the same token, couldn't we also conclude that the very affirmation of personhood in the face of the dehumanizing discourses so prevalent at the time represents in fact a legitimate combative stance? While ACT UP and other groups favored collective political action in order to, among other things, have patients recognized as co-experts on the disease and full partners in their own care, personal testimony played a part in the struggle too. When the orderlies in the operating room don't recognize Hervé as a patient because he is not wearing the proper attire, they grudgingly find themselves obligated to grant him another sort of recognition, an acknowledgment simultaneously generated by and enacting equality and the respect to which every human being is entitled. In this case, however, Hervé does not enjoy recognition as a person in the abstract—that is, in spite of his having AIDS. There is no forgetting the specific circumstances in which the confrontation is taking place. AIDS made Hervé the person that he has become, and that person with AIDS deserves to be acknowledged as such—that is, as a person and as having AIDS both at once.

At the time, prevailing public discourses (the media but also medical literature) tended to construct people with AIDS in narrative terms, making their illness the logical outcome of an unwholesome lifestyle of one kind or another. (This kind of narrative hasn't disappeared; it's only become more muted.) When the orderlies ask Hervé what he's doing there, the question is purely rhetorical; it implies that he *shouldn't* be there. The irony was probably lost on them, but hearing that he didn't belong in the hospital, for which the operating room stands as a synecdoche, must have sounded like victory.

Even though I was lucky enough to become HIV positive at a time when my life wouldn't be immediately threatened by the disease, I entered the unfamiliar universe of the hospital with the sort of baggage that comes from having spent pretty much my entire sexual existence as a gay man under the constant threat of AIDS. That stuff's bound to leave marks on a man, you know. Like everyone who was paying attention at the time, I'd heard the stories. I knew that, in the United States, in the early years, nurses sometimes wouldn't even enter a hospital room with an AIDS patient in it, that the personnel left food trays on the floor outside by the door, that bodies could remain unclaimed in the morgue for a long time because no relatives would come to collect them. I was also quite aware that, twenty-five years into the epidemic, we had come a long way and that, for the most part, such horror stories were now safely behind us. People were either better-informed or had simply grown accustomed to having that disease around. HIV clinics were just another component in any large hospital, and HIV research had become a well-respected field. Still, I entered my new life—for that's what it was—a wreck.

In the years preceding my 2006 diagnosis, I hadn't only lived through the worst times of the epidemic; I had also looked at them from a scholarly perspective. I wrote my dissertation on representations of AIDS and people with AIDS, and because it was a Ph.D. in French I was working toward, I included Guibert's work and started to write on his testimonial output while he was still alive. I went on to teach a number of Guibert's books on AIDS over the years, as well as a great many other texts about the epidemic in France. And then I stopped. Reading that stuff had begun to take an emotional toll on me, and besides, the new reality ushered in by the appearance of successful antiretroviral therapies in the second half of the 1990s bore less and less resemblance to what these critical essays and literary testimonies were trying to account for. If I wanted to keep teaching on AIDS in France, the course and its goals had to be rethought entirely. One thing I knew was that I wasn't ready to teach the epidemic as history, so I retired the course, promising myself to go back to it in due time and develop a more up-to-date version. Naturally, I never did. I was done with AIDS.

Life's complicated, though, and as I would soon learn, AIDS was not done with me. When my number came up, and even though I knew that my life would not be in any immediate danger, my inventory of HIV-related thoughts, words, and affects—my subjective archive, if you like—had remained in such pristine condition over the years, so untouched was it by changing realities about which I was actually far better-informed than the average gay man, that I ventured inside the hospital universe as if on enemy territory. Oh, I knew they wouldn't burn the chair I'd sat on or bleach the examination room after I'd left, of course, but I readied myself for a fight all the same. In retrospect, I'm not sure what I was afraid of specifically, only that a sudden sense of failure and shame had overwhelmed my defenses and left me as vulnerable to psychological abuse as my body was to infections. I went into full-blown AIDS panic mode. This was going to be a battle, I knew it, and I had to be prepared for the impending assault.

As you may have guessed, no such confrontation ever came to pass, and after a few visits, I had to admit that the nurses and social workers, and ultimately my doctor, were perfectly fine people who may in fact have my well-being in mind. Let's be clear: This happy outcome wasn't by any means a foregone conclusion. For many people living with HIV or newly infected, relations with health care professionals can remain difficult, even harrowing at times. I once met a young man who was in terrible distress in the face of a positive diagnosis that took him completely by surprise and so unfairly early in the span of his sex life. His doctor reacted by

telling him something like: "It seems to me you're implying
that you never did anything wrong." Angry and hurt, the kid
demanded to change doctors and was able to, but how many
people have the option or gumption or the sort of assured-
ness that often comes with gender, race, or class entitlement
to even ask? Others have told me of the icy reception that
met them at students' health services when they requested
an emergency post-exposure prophylaxis treatment follow-
ing what's become known as a condom accident. And that's
just people I've known in Ann Arbor, a gay-friendly college
town with a world-class research hospital.

Now, the fact that I was luckier than some didn't keep me
from complaining about a lot of things. Why did you wait
so long to contact me and schedule the first appointment
knowing what emotional turmoil I had to be going through?
Do you realize what your radio silence sounds like at my end?
Did you ever wonder about this? Oh, sure, you recognized
that, because my numbers—viral load, CD4 cell count—
were not catastrophic, other patients required your limited
attention more urgently, but how was I supposed to reach
the same dispassionate conclusion? That first time, I had to
wait an hour—a whole fucking hour!—until someone came
to get me. A guy at the check-in desk noticed that I was be-
coming increasingly agitated in the waiting room and called
a nurse who came and apologized for the delay, explaining
to me that "a difficult situation" had unexpectedly developed
with another patient and that I had to be, well, patient. A
difficult situation? What was it about? What was going on
back there? I had no idea what the inside of an HIV clinic

looked like. Should I expect to find myself in "a difficult situation" too? What did "difficult" even mean in that context? Unable to picture anything beyond my own feelings, which took over my entire mind, I concluded that the other patient was freaking out too, only way worse than I was, and that whatever was happening to him could happen to me, too. If sharing the information was supposed to reassure me, it most certainly didn't, I can tell you that. Neither did the form you gave me so that I could write my last will and testament. You know what? I never did write it; what do you think of that, huh? Oh, and about the art: Learning that one has contracted HIV is tough enough without having to deal with faux Georgia O'Keeffe pastel crap on the walls! More seriously, I complained about the unannounced presence of students during visits, which made me feel used and very close to humiliated. Was this all I was in the end—an all but anonymous object of study sitting pitifully in a boxy examination room piled between countless other identical boxy examination rooms in a gigantic university hospital? Fuck.

My reactions to the initial sequence of hospital visits, I came to realize, owed quite a bit to *Cytomegalovirus*, to that small book I hadn't opened in years but whose power to devastate had stayed with me and, as I discovered when I reread it at last, hadn't abated with time. Like Hervé, I turned a critical eye on surroundings I assumed to be hostile by definition. Like him, I stood ready to seize every occasion to reassert my dignity and defy any attempt to treat me like less than a full human being. (Not that it happened, but you know, just in case.) Sure enough, I started teaching the book again, although not in direct relation to HIV and AIDS in France. For its latest reappearance on a syllabus of mine, I included *Cytomegalovirus* in the reading list of a course that I first considered entitling "Worthlessness" but that, heeding a colleague's opinion that I could surely find something a little less uninviting for a title, I decided to rename "Unequal Lives."

So as hospital visits became fewer and further apart, and to everyone's relief including my own, I eventually calmed down and settled into my new routine. After a while I even started to look forward to catching up with people whose company I had grown to enjoy. As I explained elsewhere, my survival strategy consisted in part of reminding everyone of my status as a professor at the university and thus as my doctor's colleague as well as his patient. And because I too specialize in HIV, albeit from a humanistic perspective, the two of us have had excellent conversations over the years. During one of these chatty visits, I brought up the issue of the punitive nondisclosure laws still on the books in more than thirty of the United States in the U.S. In Michigan, for example, failure to inform a sexual partner that you are HIV positive can send you to prison regardless of actual trans-mission or even *risk* of transmission. I argued that, in addi-tion to being patently unjust, such disclosure laws are also counterproductive because they actually encourage people not to get tested so that they can't be held legally responsible for failing to reveal to their sexual partners a positive status they themselves do not know for a fact. Someone there took exception to my point and brought up the case of a man in a neighboring town who had recklessly passed on the virus to several female sexual partners without telling them that he was HIV positive: "I think that, for irresponsible guys like him, these laws make sense. Some people must be stopped before they do more harm." The town in question is poorer and has a larger African American population than the gentrified and increasingly expensive Ann Arbor, where I live and where the University of Michigan Hospital is located. I don't know whether they were talking about a black man, but at the very least, there was no mistaking the assumption of a class divide. And around Detroit, poor almost invariably means black.

That conversation made me feel very uncomfortable. It wasn't just the fact that some people from whom you'd expect better can still find arguments to defend the indefensible, or that these arguments often stem, wittingly or not, from a conservative ideology of individual responsibility that I find abhorrent; I was embarrassed that a health care professional told me that story at all. Clearly, no confidentiality rules were ever breached. Yet—and I could be wrong, of course—I had the distinct feeling that not everyone would have been deemed a suitable recipient for this information. I was *in*, now, I had made it into a rarefied circle that the possibly black serial fucker who deserved to be locked up could never dream of reaching. Suddenly I didn't like being there anymore—in, I mean. As an HIV-positive gay man—

worse, as an unreconstructed HIV-positive, working-class, immigrant gay son of an immigrant—I didn't deserve to be there. I *shouldn't* have been there. Part of me, I thought, belonged with the other guy, the one who had to be removed from society. I felt a little disgusted with myself. I was looking for the sort of respect to which every human being is entitled, and I appeared to have achieved something different altogether, something that not every human being is entitled to and that, as a result, we may not even want to call respect at all.

If you bring together Hervé's observation that "You have to make them respect you" and the proposition he made to the bitchy nurse that they both wear a transparent gown and walk hand-in-hand to surgery, it becomes apparent that, for him, respect and equality cannot exist separately. Respect makes manifest one's recognition of the universal principle of human equality. My mistake, however, was to let my initial desire to make a claim for equality in the name of the overarching ideal of justice lead me instead to a far baser affirmation of social privilege. (I'm not sure this was entirely my fault, really. Power dynamics, especially when enforced by weighty institutions such as "the university" or "the hospital," do not lend themselves willingly to the sort of durable transformation that personal behavior is ever likely to effect. I don't believe that Guibert, as successful a writer as he was, envisioned that major changes would result from his small acts of resistance.) It wasn't until my interlocutors inadvertently made it obvious that they considered me *their* equal but not that of the other, "bad" HIV patient that I realized how far I'd strayed. Relative equality is no equality at all. I wanted respect and what I got instead was respectability.

Thinking of recognition and lack thereof, I don't remember when it happened exactly, around the thirtieth anniversary for sure, but it suddenly dawned on me that AIDS had entered the realm of history. The signs have been unmistakable. In 2011, for example, Broadway saw a triumphant revival of Larry Kramer's 1985 play *The Normal Heart*, a self-aggrandizing jeremiad on the early years of the epidemic and the folly of queens. A high-profile HBO movie followed three years later. Hell! It even had Julia Roberts in it. Another Broadway revival, that of James Lapine and William Finn's AIDS musical *Falsettos* (1992), has been announced, while London is, as I'm writing this, enjoying the return of a British play, Kevin Elyot's *My Night with Reg* (1994). Given the extraordinary theatrical output that the AIDS crisis produced in the English-speaking world, it is safe to assume that more may be coming our way—until of course people become tired of stories about AIDS.

Biographies and autobiographies of important figures of the terrible years have also begun to come out regularly—Vito Russo, John Weir, Sean Strub, David Wojnarowicz, Michael Callen. . . . Two documentaries on the history of ACT UP–New York appeared at almost the same time in 2012: Jim Hubbard's uncompromising *United in Anger* and David France's Oscar-nominated *How to Survive a Plague*. And on a recent trip to Paris, I discovered a striking number of memoirs by friends, lovers, and siblings of people lost to the epidemic (including one by a former lover of Guibert's). France being France, narrative literature played a central role in bringing AIDS to public attention there; Guibert was the first author to reach that large an audience and the only one to attain canonical status, but there were many others. Most of them have been forgotten, but back then they enjoyed a remarkable degree of visibility in the media, notably in the wake of Guibert's success. It seems only fitting that literature should once more testify to the ravages of AIDS, this time as history.

Thirty years. Wasn't it thirty years after the liberation of the camps that Claude Lanzmann began work on his monumental film *Shoah?* Yes, after thirty years, the time has come to tell the story.

It was with mixed emotions that I greeted the realization that, in Western countries, AIDS had become history. With the constant development of new successful treatments, and now prophylaxis, the worst times of the epidemic seem to have gone for good, and I find it reassuring that the prevailing attitude among some of the surviving witnesses is to remember, to document, and to tell of the struggle that took place in the not-so-distant past. Anyone who teaches HIV and AIDS, at least aspects of the epidemic other than strictly medical, has had to confront his or her students' ignorance of what happened in earlier years other than the fact that a lot of people died and that many had to face some kind of bigotry. But beyond that, what?

Younger audiences may have seen the Oscar-winning

Hollywood film *Dallas Buyers Club*, about a community-run pharmacy that distributes HIV drugs smuggled from Mexico and unapproved in the United States. If they did, what they saw was the story of an HIV-positive heterosexual man who overcomes his homophobia thanks to his friendship with a sacrificial transgender prostitute whose narrative function suggests a queer version of the "magic Negro." The fact that in reality these pharmacies and underground networks were overwhelmingly run by gay people has simply been erased from history in favor of a mostly true but atypical story about a straight anti-hero badly in need of redemption.

Around the same time, the local art house that had shown *Dallas Buyers Club* for an extended, successful run brought *How to Survive a Plague* to Ann Arbor. The night I went to see the movie, the smaller screening room in which it played was disappointingly empty, or just about. There couldn't have been more than a dozen people in there, and I wouldn't be too surprised if all of them, like me, already knew much of the story the movie had to tell. By contrast, a showing of *United in Anger* a few days later filled the much larger main theater with hundreds of undergraduates who, needless to say, were required to attend by their professors. The Q&A with the director after the screening may not have provided a statistically significant sample, obviously, but the reactions that a few students expressed in public—something like, "I had no idea this happened, and wow! It's so amazing and so inspiring!"—were probably quite telling and certainly squared with what I keep witnessing in my classes. The historical patina these events have acquired may obscure the ongoing realities of the epidemic, but if students get to see footage of police brutality against AIDS activists fighting for their lives and manage to make connections with the more familiar images of the civil rights struggle, it is definitely cause for rejoicing, for decades will pass before the fight against AIDS makes it into their American history books—if it ever does.

But just as racist discrimination and violence haven't ended with the election of the first African American president of the United States, it would be just as unwise to mistake progress for victory on the HIV front. Almost twenty years after the development of life-prolonging drugs, still well over 15,000 people die of AIDS-related causes in the United States every year. And if you're under the impression that bigotry and discrimination against people living with HIV are a thing of the past, think again. I'm not just talking about social interactions or sexual rejection either; as I said, more than thirty states in the U.S. have laws that, in one way or another, criminalize HIV positivity. While activists have been working tirelessly to have these laws overturned, people would be shocked to learn that someone who never even infected anyone could end up in jail for years and on a sex-offender registry for life, making keeping a job and a roof over their heads nearly impossible for a great number of them. This is not history; this is the America we live in today, and most people have no idea all this is happening.

The ambivalence that often characterizes historical memory is not new, and one could argue that, in that respect, early AIDS activism has been subjected to contrary forces not so different from those that the civil rights struggle of the 1950s and 1960s has been facing. To put it succinctly: Memorialize and forget it. By that I mean, memorialize the past and its heroes, but forget the present and those who are still in the trenches. The big difference, of course, is that the memory of AIDS activism hasn't reached far beyond very small circles of academics and community activists. Nationally, the genocidal moment of the AIDS crisis has recessed into oblivion without its ever having been fully acknowledged in the first place.

Incidentally, I didn't mention *Shoah* by accident. This documentary on the Holocaust, as is well known, doesn't make any use of archival footage in its nine-and-a-half-hour running time—no bulldozers pushing piles of corpses into mass graves, no haunting faces of survivors staring back at us, none of that. One of the many reasons why *Shoah* has had such an impact is that the debate on representations of the Holocaust it triggered has not yet concluded. Lanzmann's decision to shoot his film on location in the present day, in villages near Chelmno or at Treblinka's old train station, for example, reveals the past's disturbing persistence and the events' stubborn resistance to remaining safely contained by certain historiography, official memory, or any other means of telling the facts the better to erase them from memory. Is this, then, what we are currently witnessing with regard to the AIDS crisis? If so, how does this sort of forgetfulness work and why has it come about? Conversely, what is it about Hervé Guibert's hospital diary, written in 1991, that makes republishing it a quarter-century later feel so vital?

A student of mine—a young, intelligent heterosexual woman—once told me that for people of her generation, HIV and AIDS couldn't be further from their minds. She'd been reading Guibert's second volume dealing with his illness, *The Compassion Protocol*, for our class, and the whole thing sounded like the distant past to her. It *is* the distant past, there's no denying that, but, I thought, shouldn't she and her peers feel at least a little bit concerned about contracting a virus that is still very much around and liable to, if not kill you, at least tether you for the rest of your life to serious and expensive treatments whose long-term effects are not yet known? But I'm not one to lecture twenty-year-olds about long-term effects, of this or anything else; I'm a teacher, I know better. To be fair, one could argue that middle- and upper-class straight kids have indeed remained far less likely to become infected with HIV than young gay men, especially young gay men of color. Yet, even within more vulnerable populations, it seems that the combination of medical progress and the simple passing of time has relegated concerns about HIV to secondary status, if that.

Time doesn't move along unaccompanied, however, and people don't lose interest collectively, just like that, as though unmoored from larger cultural and political forces within which interests arise and recede. In truth, HIV hasn't disappeared from people's personal lives; it has merely been kept at bay, and uneasily so at that. Male–male sex ads and hookup profiles on hookup sites, for example, routinely make mention of HIV, if only for exclusionary purposes, to require that potential partners be negative. More tragically, I have witnessed first-hand the distress that often comes with the diagnosis even today. If we, as a culture, don't think about AIDS so much anymore—that is, if we don't think about it other than negatively, as a cause for rejection or psychological trauma rather than as a call to action—it is very likely that we've been induced not to by certain public discourses. Gays and lesbians in particular have been encouraged to care about other and apparently more pressing issues. The recent historicization of the AIDS crisis, it seems to me, cannot be separated from the political agenda set by mainstream LGBT advocacy groups.

As you are reading these pages, the U.S. Supreme Court has probably already legalized same-sex marriage all over the country. I'm guessing that you're happy about that too, as indeed I am. Equal rights under the law are nothing to be sneezed at, after all. And even though it's all a bit far now, we may remember that from the very beginning of the recent struggle for the legal recognition of same-sex couples, before domestic partnership made room for full marriage equality, the tragedies wrought by the AIDS epidemic took center stage in the rhetoric. They brought to the cause the sort of emotional punch more likely to sway minds in the larger culture at the early stages of the fight than the more ethical, but also less tangible, principle of equality. I saw it happen in France and I saw it happen here in the United States. The stories were the same, they were true, and they were horrific. Lovers with no hospital visitation rights; friends who provided care from the start sidelined at the last minute by greedy relatives nobody even knew of; life partners expelled from apartments because only one person could sign the lease and that lease happened to be in the name of the other man, now dead. The inhumane treatment of people with AIDS and of the friends who cared physically, psychologically, and materially for them occupied a central part in the legalization rhetoric and contributed its fair share to rallying a sympathetic public to the cause of marriage equality.

This is no longer the case now that the right to marry has reached the courts and draws support primarily by relying on the rhetoric of equality as a principle of law rather than as an answer to people's concrete needs. The question of visitation rights hasn't vanished from this rhetoric; what has vanished, or at least faded, is the issue's link to HIV and AIDS. The purpose of equality, it seems, is no longer the full respect of vulnerable flesh-and-blood human beings but unimpeded access to services for all. And this is far from negligible, of course; don't think I'm being dismissive. In fact, one could argue that the amazing progress in the treatment of HIV that, for many, has transformed the disease into a manageable chronic condition explains why hospital visitation rights and medical decision making for spouses seem self-evident whether you're gay or not. If we no longer bring up the tragedies of the past, it is precisely because they are of the past. They have done their job, as it were. In other words, it's all good. Or, rather, it would be if, perhaps, we hadn't mistaken respect for respectability and reduced to a simple matter of legal equality the universal principle that all human beings are worth the same.

HIV does remain an important preoccupation for a lot

of people (with 50,000 new infections a year in the United States alone, how could it not?), some of them involved enough to do something about it. More often than not, however, well-meaning efforts don't reach beyond information and prevention. I once asked an administrator of the Spectrum Center, the University of Michigan's office serving LGBT students, what they were doing to help students with HIV. The response came as if on cue: "We offer regular testing for free; we also organize information sessions on prevention with . . . ." "This is great for students who are HIV negative," I replied, "but this isn't what I'm asking. I would like to know what you're doing for students who already *are* HIV positive." "Oh. . . ." She froze for a second. She hadn't even heard my question. I couldn't blame her, and the reaction didn't surprise me. For most people with the purest of motives, prevention remains the primary concern when thinking about HIV in daily life.

This anecdote reveals a far more complex dynamic than, for example, that of sexual rejection. In a good mood, you can forgive guys you'd like to sleep with for being misinformed, silly, even for being outright jerks who harm others for no good reason. But in this case, my interlocutors were people who were on my side, whose business it was to be on my side. And the thought hadn't crossed their minds. To be fair, they recognized the problem and were immediately receptive to my suggestions. I'm happy to say that a support group for students living with HIV is now active. I'm less happy to say that when the Center's director searched the websites of similar campus LGBT offices for models to emulate on its own, she didn't find anything that addressed the needs of HIV-positive students. Our students must be protected from HIV infections, and we all agree on that, but those among them who are living with HIV, it seems, do not exist at all. Between prevention and treatment, no room exists to *live* with HIV.

Thankfully, other activists and advocates of various stripes are still on the front lines, reframing HIV issues in relation to changing circumstances and insisting that we can understand the epidemic only in relation to the larger social conditions from which it draws. Today, HIV advocacy may focus simultaneously on so-called sex crimes in general, not just disclosure laws; or it may connect the continuing epidemic with the equally maddening problem of mass incarceration that has increased African American communities' vulnerability to HIV. It has always been the case that the contours of the AIDS epidemic have duplicated those of social inequality and exclusion, but the mainstreaming of rights-oriented gay politics has increasingly relegated HIV to the sidelines. Indeed, when marriage equality became the priority, it probably seemed wiser to avoid potentially damaging mentions of sex, crime, and the continuing oppression of people of color. And what better way to forget HIV than to dismiss people with HIV?

If you hang out in certain gay circles, for example, in particular around men in my age group who remember the early, darker years of the AIDS crisis, you probably have heard someone exclaim something like, "How stupid do you have to be to become infected now?" usually followed by "Doesn't everyone know how to protect themselves already?" Yeah, well, things often don't turn out as planned. And that too we can hear often. Or we could if we paid attention, but why listen to people we've already decided are not intelligent? Who cares what stupid things they have to say?

Coming from gay men, who should know better, this attitude sounds especially callous, disturbing even, because when they call others irresponsible they betray their own desire to absolve themselves of any residual duty to share in the continuing burden of the epidemic. Morally, I find it particularly repugnant because it blames and abandons vulnerable people; politically, it comes perilously close to the same neoliberal dogma on individual responsibility that underlies the criminalization of nondisclosure.

I'm not telling these stories for the pleasure of venting outrage, as you can imagine, but because they seem to me emblematic of a broader, if unacknowledged, tendency to sideline the issue of HIV by invalidating the very people who live with it and to dismiss them as unintelligent, uninteresting, or outlying throwbacks to what we now consider ancient history. But can't we also make the parallel claim that it was because of a perceived political need to make AIDS ancient history that people with HIV had to be delegitimized? Either way, seropositivity no longer provides a recognized subject-position from which to think, to make knowledge, to speak, let alone to act politically in the world we currently live in. And because of the relational nature of subjecthood, a subject can emerge from its recognition only as such. No recognition, no subject; no subject, no thought; no thought, no words; no words, no recognition. Removed from any process of signification, being HIV positive literally no longer means anything.

In the face of such erasure, Hervé Guibert's account of his daily struggles for recognition, one dessert spoon at a time, sounds as urgent and as compelling as it ever did. As the fight against the epidemic has taken a much more painstaking and unspectacular form than what groups like ACT UP once offered, and as the disease has receded from public view, it has become more necessary than ever for people living with HIV to resist their erasure from everyday life and be acknowledged. *Cytomegalovirus*, far from depicting the struggle against HIV and AIDS as a matter of individual heroics, reminds us instead that at the very core of this struggle stands a full person made more vulnerable by a web of exclusionary social forces. So let's be clear, HIV has never been and will never be a respectable disease. To begin with, it will largely remain associated with undesirable categories of people, as new infection trends indicate. And the image of two men taking marriage vows in front of a minister and their loved ones may momentarily distract from actual homosexual acts, but HIV can't perform that trick. As Guibert's example reminds us, people with HIV are not treated unequally so much as unjustly. Their mistreatment or outright dismissal constitutes not simply an attack on their social or legal status but rather a denial of their humanity. Against that, respectability is of little help. "You have to make them respect you," remember, "or they flatten you." No Supreme Court decision alone, as welcome, fair, and necessary as it is, will ever compel respect. But who knows, a dessert spoon just might.

Cytomegalovirus
A Hospitalization Diary

September 17

Vision in my right eye is shot: difficulty reading. Listen to music: not yet deaf.

September 18

A young woman with a very beautiful, made-up face, who looked a little Asian, lying unconscious on an abandoned stretcher in a radiology corridor, very red lips, and something on her uncovered neck which I at first thought was a wound, as if someone had tried to cut her throat, but which apparently turned out to be a long smear of lipstick.

Waiting behind a window before the abdominal ultrasound: you can see the hospital visitors descend the esca-
lator and move toward one ward or another. Many men
of all ages talking to themselves, agitated. The old ones
in pajamas and robes. The young ones often bare-chested
under an open shirt or jacket.

Cytomegalovirus! Hospitalization.

Lenses right on the retina.

I'm afraid they'll make me sleep in paper sheets, under a
synthetic blanket.

The will to live—marvelous or sickening?

They used to tell me: "You have beautiful eyes," or "You
have beautiful lips"; now, nurses tell me, "You have beautiful veins." The doctor, a young woman with a foreign
accent who took the abdominal ultrasound, tells her
assistant, who is leaning over her shoulder in front of the
screen: "Look at how beautiful that is!" And to me: "You
have a truly exceptional and very rare interior configura-
tion. We are also going to take some pictures for ourselves."

September 19

The sheets are not made out of paper, the blanket is not
synthetic: good, old, used hospital sheets, a real wool blanket, from a hospital or barracks.

No shower in the room (now I realize that this terror of a communal shower, one which has no privacy, stems from my childhood), no towels in the bathroom. H.G. tells me that the nurse's aide almost choked with indignation when he asked for one. Paper towels. B. and H.G. insisted on buying me a real towel. They also brought back a small spoon, a little box of sugar (my Briard whole milk yogurts in glass jars, which are in a refrigerator with my room number—365—on them, in a small room next door, "the best in the world," says B.). They also brought me black grapes, my good friends.

The window allows permanent viewing from the corridor into the room. I don't say anything. B. says: "All you have to do is push the closet door."

Young, vaguely Asian intern, extremely kind and competent. She says she knows Claudette Dumouchel, I tell her, laughing, "I promise I won't write *Le protocole compassionnel #2*, so you can relax, we can have a nice relationship." We joke. She asks me if I have written lately, and I say yes: "Something which has no connection to AIDS and which I've never done before, a very physical love story between a man and woman, what's more, a very exotic novel, that's why I went to Bora Bora!" We ask each other what we like about our respective professions, that's good. I ask her: "If, for one reason or another, they hadn't detected the cytomegalovirus right away, how long would it have taken me to lose my eye; would it have taken months, weeks, days?"

"Days," she answers. We may not be able to save it as it is, we'll see!

Weakness, fatigue, I leaf through the papers, no desire to listen to the radio that I asked H.G. to bring. No time to get bored, always a caregiver passing by, or the telephone.

T. asked what I see from my windows, I move around the room telling him: "A beltway on the outskirts of town, a little forest, a truck rental and repair shop, the hospital parking lot, some trees. And, in the distance, Paris."

Dietitian (I asked to see her when I arrived) also kind and competent. A half hour of back-and-forth questioning. I gorged myself this evening, on the tray I found the menu typed on the word processor, I hid it under the dish of grapes so I could copy it. Better than Air France.

Start an intravenous line. They hook me up to an old crock that doesn't even move. This severely reduces my ability to move around the room. I try to do a lot of things in the same place (pissing and brushing my teeth, for example) so as not to have to make too many trips. But I've already asked two nurses to scrounge up an IV pole that moves. I'll keep asking until I get it.

At dinner: only one spoon for both the soup and the farmer's cheese, I ask, on principle, if they expect me to clean it with my tongue? Special treatment.

Obviously can't find the buzzer, always been awkward. And—I don't know how—I tangle the intravenous tube around the pole, soon I'll only be able to move a few inches.

They warn that it will hurt, they prick a very large needle in a painful spot, almost at the wrist, to leave the upper veins free for blood draws. I asked the intern to have the kindness to instruct that they only draw blood if absolutely necessary, and not on the slightest whim, as they often do in hospitals.

Writing is also a way of giving rhythm to time and a way to pass it.

I'm waiting for them to do the IV (I love adopting the pro lingo—with cytomegalovirus, they won't do an LP, lumbar puncture, on me), I'll get it lying down, it is eight in the evening, I'm tired. It's been a long day. Till tomorrow.

I get up to jot down some phrases that swim through my head, or else they'll haunt me until tomorrow. The cries of suffering which come from nearby rooms are almost more heart-wrenching than one's own suffering. The neighbor screams, the nurse tells him, "Open your mouth wide," I wonder what she can possibly be doing to him.

Today, I may have made the acquaintance of the room in which I will die. I don't like it yet.

You have to wait between five and ten minutes after buzzing, you have the impression that the nurses go on a one-shift wildcat strike so they can steal away on roller-skates to party at the *La Rumba* nightclub in the Auchan superstore.

The room hasn't been disinfected or even swept: old bandages under the bed. Proof. The nurse to whom I mentioned it hurries to gather everything to throw it out. She says, "It's disgusting." And I say, "You're not going to mark it as evidence."

D. always said that M., who was going to die anyway, died much more brutally because he was hospitalized in a room that hadn't been disinfected so as to keep the hallway clear. Hospital illness.

When a nurse installs my IV, I can't help but think it may be water, "since in any case, he's going to croak," and remember the three lesbian nurses of Tübingen who liquidated old geezers by sticking a little spoon under their tongues and flooding their lungs.

The sleeping pills seem like amphetamines!

Z. told me that she would bring me a soft light; personally, I love this leaden, blinding white neon.

The War Diary of Babel: if I lose my eye, it will be one of the last books I opened. This diary should also be a war diary.

On the admission form this afternoon, three options: "stretcher," "wheelchair," "can walk." I still can.

Midnight. I got up to pee, they would have woken me up anyway to take my temperature, my blood pressure. The kindly nurse, the one who deplores my non-moving pole and with whom I can relax and have a nice time, installed a hep-lock in me (after the "vein protector"), the instrument I needed so I could move around, that I had been asking for since six o'clock of the little crabby blond nurse, who told me it didn't exist here. The heroes and villains, just like in fairy tales.

There's an eye at stake.

"Open your mouth! Did you hear me?" asks the big nurse. "Yes, what are they doing?" Answer: a mouth rinse. The Tübingen nurses.

They gab away all night without lowering their voices in the room next to mine, about salaries and the cost of living. I'll have to call my accountant one of these days.

A hospital stay is like a long voyage with an uninterrupted parade of people, of deliveries, or of rituals, to pass the time. There isn't even any more night.

Hospitals are hell.

Much later at night, they lower their voices a little, even they are tired.

Screams in the next room, like bellowing cows. No way to get some sleep.

September 20

They always wake you up at seven o'clock in the morning to stick a thermometer under your armpit. At eight, five tubes of blood taken through the hep-lock. The morning nurse seems nice. There are pearls, and there are swine. Yellow sun through the window.

One could write a humorous dictionary of AIDS term: the candidate is a fungus that declares he's running so he can take over your throat, your esophagus, your stomach, and eat them.

Beautiful sunshine. The IV pole does not move around, of course, the breakfast table is broken, and the toilet flush takes five minutes to stop its racket, everyone knows that.

Alarming news from V. yesterday before leaving for the hospital. His Brazilian girlfriend tells me, "Wait, I'll go see." She comes back whispering, "V. is in no condition to talk. But call back, it'll make him happy, he needs it so much." I say, "Is it his morale?" She says: "You know, he pops so many pills, he's in horrible shape." I think he's started to shoot up, he mentioned it to me the last two times we saw each other. A long time ago, I was the one who wanted to shoot up, and he's the one who didn't want to. When he proposed it the last few times, I'm the one who said no.

I ring the bell again because in the hall I heard a nurse who had just left my room tell a colleague (in a mocking tone) "He said that his IV doesn't flow quickly enough and that it was starting to hurt him." I call back just to say, "I never said that."

The neighbor's howling. Either he's very delicate, or it's very painful. I'm unfortunately leaning toward the second hypothesis. Maybe soon I'll be the one screaming.

The IV didn't flow because the kind and pretty intern made a prescription error.

No time to go down to buy the paper.

I snitched to the authorities about the state of filth in my room after they told me it was "ready." This morning the intern, a rather young man, told me, "I assure you that the person here before you didn't have anything serious, just a little vascular trouble."

Nighttime here: fighting against a steam-roller advancing, I dare not say blindly, without its driver. If you don't resist, if you don't run, it will crush you. Under the circumstances, it's better to remain a human being than a bloody pancake.

At first, you get a big punch in the gut, it's sadness, despair, you forbid yourself to cry. Then, you try to find reasons to sustain the will to live. Getting euphoric is dangerous, because from there, you risk falling apart.

They just discovered that the IV also did not flow because the needle, which had been poorly inserted last night, had come out half way, producing a small hematoma that has already practically resorbed.

This risk of destroying someone, of causing someone who really needs their job to lose it (if they didn't need the job they wouldn't do it, or they might do it only out of a sense of vocation), not even the notion of vengeance, but simply the ethical notion that everyone is expected to do their jobs well. The writer also can be destroyed, if suddenly he starts writing shit or stuff that's unacceptable.

These planes taking off: I try to see them through the window.

I must admit I have trouble reading even a newspaper article. Writing, less difficult.

The nurse who came, almost clandestinely, to install the hep-lock at midnight dropped it on the dirty floor. Since she wears gloves, she can't really grasp objects. She brings back another one, or at least I hope it's another one, and she says: "This time I better not drop it, it's the last one on the ward."

Professor D., assistant head of the ward, came by; I ask him: "So, would you like my wife to send a registered letter to the head of the ward?" "No, not now," he answers without trembling. I am growing to like this bear better and better with every visit.

I can't easily tell the time on my watch; I must admit I'm having trouble despite my eye because this Swatch was already pretty illegible.

Since childhood, this obsession with eyes, like a backward premonition. And the novel written in '83 and '84: *Des aveugles* (*Of the Blind*)!

Today: "Lunch—1 normal (I write it down). Greek style mushrooms. Skate fish sautéed in butter. English style taters. Farmer's cheese 40% fat. Plums. Bread 50 grams." We all know about this mysterious, imperious and boring mania that hospital patients have of describing for their already sickened visitors everything they stuffed down (promise, you won't know tonight's menu, unless it's something really extravagant). Yesterday's first menu that I hid so I could copy it has disappeared: either someone stole it from me—but I believe in a less paranoid cause—or I hid it too well and I can't find it anymore (under my blue hat?), or a nurse took it by accident when she opened the curtains.

HHC: home health care, but at the earliest in two weeks.

Tuesday they'll surgically insert a port-a-cath [*porte-à-cath*] in my torso, to give my vein a rest, because the antiviral is very toxic.

"What, no hep-lock in the ward?" the professor asks the nurse, more pale than before. "Did you ask in pulmonary?" "Yes, they don't have any either." "So call cardiology."

You have to make them respect you right away, it's exhausting, a test of wills that lasts one or even several days and nights. They want you to lose, they count on wearing you down. Then, according to the situation, they respect or they flatten you.

They are an army of poor women who stick together. The men, the minority, are either bosses or flunkies.

What's more, on a whim, July 13 (two months ago) I stopped taking the antidepressants. It just kept getting worse: dry mouth, palpitations, stronger and stronger doses, I told myself: Let's try, it's now or never. I'm on the island of Elba, I'm not writing (writing for me is always also a kind of antidepressant), but there's silence, the ocean, the presence and screeching of the birds, they should be my tranquilizers. In any case, if it's hell, I'll take some right away because I have enough to last my entire stay. Not only was it not hell, but, after a little paranoid attack, my morale was better.

This evening I'll leave the window open to hear the noise of the traffic on the beltway, in the hopes of muffling a bit the neighbor's screams and the night nurses' idle gossip.

Actually, they aren't airplanes, but helicopters that land on the hospital roof with seriously injured patients. Between two weeks and three months ago I flew in a helicopter, in good health, to Bora Bora. Takeoff and landing were sublimely smooth, unreal, not to mention the blue and green hues from above.

I called my parents, happy on vacation, to tell them I'd be hospitalized for a few days, "to take care of some crap," without going into the details, refusing to tell them where and forbidding them to call T. and C. every day, as they threatened to do.

This diary, which should last two weeks, may stop any day due to absolute discouragement.

Left the curtains open this evening to see the twilight, in blue and pink tones, during the IV, and the moon, veiled with a halo, hypnotic.

I ask the orderly what the difference is between an orderly and a nurse, and she tells me: "The nurse deals with all the drugs, IV, blood draws. Me, I'm here to change your sheets, or if you want a 'pistolet.'" I ask (with false innocence): "So I can shoot myself?" And she says, thinking I'm crazy, "No, if you want to pee without getting up." I say, "I can still get up."

There are airplanes after all, and even bats, night has fallen, I'm still waiting for the IV. The psychologist just told me, with a diabolical smile, motionless, made up like the mask of a Japanese Nô performer: "But one doesn't sleep in the hospital, one doesn't rest in the hospital!"

For the last few minutes, there's been a massive yellow Temesta (2.5 mg) and a capsule of Prozac, an antidepressant, on my table. I don't know if I'll take them.

The nurse who came to give me my IV sings the praises of eye injections, saying, "What's better, an injection in the eye (personally, I know I could never stand that), or to become completely blind?" So I can dream sweet dreams? See you tomorrow?

The moon moves slowly from one window to the next. A zone in-between where it becomes invisible.

The sheets stained with blood. The hep-lock is disgusting when it's pulled out after each use: a long, very fine and flexible plastic tube stained with black, half-coagulated blood. But it's better than that immovable pole. Pain in the lower back. Bruised vein.

September 21

Beautiful sky but it won't be beautiful for long, unless it's too early for the sun. Even roosters! It's almost like being in the country! They didn't wake me at seven like yesterday. I woke up by myself, despite the yellow Temesta. I slept, I feel rested, it's a nice feeling.

The big, friendly, gawky made-up woman, who's always lucky with men, stubborn as a mule: she programmed my IV to stop at midnight for reasons of convenience. It stopped at midnight on the dot, even though they still pretend not to be able to control it. The open window worked relatively well, but around three in the morning the traffic slows down, and my neighbor screamed again. I waited for the waves of trucks.

I don't know if, with this hospitalization diary, I'm doing any good or harm. I have the impression that there are writers who do good (Hamsun, Walser, Handke, and even paradoxically Bernhard in the energy of his genius for writing), and those who do evil (Sade obviously, Dostoevsky?). Now I'd rather belong to the first group.

Week-end. No one. Wide open doors, as if all the rooms were empty and their occupants had left for a great communal picnic. Buzzing a few minutes, ten minutes, fifteen minutes does no good.

I decided to take the first Prozac yesterday at midnight, after more than a year's interruption due to "tolerance" [*échappement*] for the product (it's the psychiatric term: it no longer had an effect on me). T. was against it, with a logic I understood (vicious circle, stronger and stronger products, fight alone, the second day in the hospital is always the worst, etc.). M. was for it, H., my friend the psychiatrist, was really for it, and the intern called to the rescue, without whom I could not obtain the product, was also for it. I too become for it in time, although hesitating until midnight. I thought: Prozac takes ten days to take effect, which will be exactly the time necessary to verify if there's been an effect on the fundus of the eye, when they'll tell me if the treatment worked or not, if I've already lost one eye and risk losing the other, unless they try injections, and then I know that, if this should happen, I would need some chemical assistance not to crack up.

There's the one you see for the first time, and who brings you, in two minutes, the indispensable inclined table that you've asked for fifty times in two days to twenty different nurses. Once and for all, they decided to say that there weren't any, they must think it's less of a pain for them than to push a little table down the hall. There's dried vomit under my new table, but it isn't broken.

"If the vein bursts," the nurse says, "we'll prick higher. We always start low and move up." So the vein may burst.

A bursting vein could be very beautiful: a jet stream that spurts everywhere, a deep red "blood-works," a blood bouquet. As soon as I'm thinking of it, my blood starts to boil in the plastic tubes. No, it's not a burst vein, but a blood reflux.

I went out of my room for the first time this morning, after having shaved (I cut myself, which never happens: I may have to use the Gillette Sensor which B. talks up so much) and put on my blue hat. I met no one, except the intern, who told me I was right to take the Prozac. I went out just to buy *Libération*. The newsstand is closed Saturday and Sunday. T. is supposed to stop by to see me this afternoon.

Today is the second and last day of "palu" treatments, two bitter tablets which cause stomach cramps, to be taken every six hours.

No more IV pole at all: the duty nurse went to find one
for me.

I refused to let my sister come see me today. I hesitate to
call V. back.

I'm not saying I'd like to become blind, there are situations
so desperate that one tries to take advantage of them, but
it's something I'm not familiar with, and I always love to
slip into known situations, no matter the consequences.

D. was saying that M., a few days before death, in the
intensive care unit, must have developed an exceptional
relationship with the doctor on call. They talked together
all night. I think that inevitably, even if one doesn't want to
develop, or pretends not to want to develop, any personal
relationship and prefers to deal with issues through the
technological framework of illness, as has been the case
between me and my doctor for more than a year, the doctor and patient develop a personal rapport, almost a feeling
of closeness. M.'s night doctor has up till now kept all his
secrets in anonymity and silence.

My doctor came to see me just now. He announced that if
the port-a-cath installation goes well under local anesthesia
in the operating room, they would start the administra-
tive procedures that would permit me to be hospitalized
at home as soon as possible, and sooner than anticipated

(simultaneously I thought: Great! and Shit! my diary won't continue for two weeks).

Last night, she came back, small, yellow skin, visibly un-happy, to take my blood pressure, and I told her: "Would you allow me to point out to you, Miss or Mrs., that I found you to have acted rather badly toward me the other evening, on a human, an ethical and professional level?" "What do you mean by that?" she asked, frozen, trauma-tized. "Well, this: you must know by now that an AIDS patient, thus someone who is very weak and tired, must come to terms with the shock of learning that he risks losing his sight. You must also understand the shock of being hospitalized for two weeks. So you act like a jerk, you tell me that the hep-lock that I've been asking for in order to free myself of this pole that doesn't move not only is not available on the ward but it doesn't even exist, that it's a fabrication of my mind, and that I will have to remain two weeks like a prisoner at his task, chained to a pole that keeps me from moving, even in my own room." She denies it: "I never said that." "We can check it on the flow chart, I didn't have any fever last night, I wasn't that delirious." She become so yellow and transfixed that I tried to make a joke of it, saying, "You must have spoken Chinese (the yellow of her skin?) and I some other language, that's why we didn't understand each other. I thought: look out for that one, she's mean, but I hope in a few days to be able to say, 'it turns out she's really kind.' And you, I hope, will think

one day, 'I thought that guy was a whiner, but not at all!'"
She now refuses to take care of me, and sent in her place
the big, petulant brunette who sings the praises of ocular
injections.

My doctor also, yesterday, uttered the word. I only had
to say, "Well, it's something I decided not to transgress
[*transgresser*]."

Empty this evening, as if I had fought a boxing match for
two days and nights while ill, against about fifty people
presumably in good health. The moon delayed showing
itself this evening, and then it was only a spark in the
veiled sky. Thanks to the kindness of a nurse, I was able
to have my IV dose at eight in the evening, and to have
it last only an hour as scheduled. It is nine-thirty. I have
just finished drinking a carton of whole milk with a
straw, the kind they give children in school. On the carton
was written "For school use only." I hope to have time
to rest.

September 22

This morning I tried to find Turner's or Constable's water-
colors in the veiled sky. At times, there were some. Then
the sky cleared up so much that it merely became a sky fit
for a beautiful day in the Paris suburbs. But all skies are
beautiful. If I could have, I would have tried to collect
paintings of skies, but they are rare.

When American billionaires have trouble with their eyes and risk losing them, they travel to Colombia, which has the best eye surgeons in the world. A poor drunk fellow had rolled into a ditch a few days earlier and, dead drunk, rolled into it a second time. He wakes up. Black hole. Everything is dark, he can't see anything, touches his eyes and finds out they've been bandaged. Another black hole in his memory: vague voices and car trips, maybe a hospital. His mother has come to grips with the fact: they stole her son's eyes. She files a complaint, orders an investigation. They declare that the eye extraction could only have been performed by a very high-level surgeon because he left the very fine nerves around the eyes, which easily could have been ruined, intact. He did a masterful job. From the accounts of the boy whose eyes were stolen, since his memory is coming back, they think they've discovered the hospital where the crime took place. But the whole ophthalmology staff has been replaced, and the others can't be found anywhere. They all left to live somewhere in the United States, with enough cash to last them the rest of their lives.

In the nurses' lounge, the nurses vie to tell their patient stories, because each one of course has an even more outrageous one to tell than the others'.

The conviviality of rotations, of shift changes. Some are going to bed, others are just getting out of bed, out of the metro or bus. "How's it going, hon? Get some rest. Got time for a bite together?"

The hospital room is an insidious cocoon that, little by little, makes the real space outside frightening, even the hallway.

I shaved twice this morning, without realizing it at first, I found the blade worn out. Sunday morning. No newspapers. Nothing to do. At the hospital, M. really wanted friends to bring him *Libé*.

The songs from a televised mass coming from a neighboring room. I go down to get a cup of coffee.

My usual awkwardness, my new weakness, plus the big catheter in my vein make it difficult even to open a packet of instant coffee.

The nursing supervisor came into my room yesterday, while I was talking to the intern. "So, what's going on? Will you tell me?" I answer her that there's really nothing to say about the hygienic conditions under which I moved into this room. "Besides that," I said, "they finally found me a breakfast tray that doesn't spill everything into the bed, but they still haven't changed my broken IV pole." She immediately takes the pole out of the room, you can hear her in the hall talking to herself as she pulls the thing: "Ah! If I don't do it myself, nothing gets done, I'll bring you one in two minutes." This evening, the nurse didn't have a pole in my room with which to do the IV. She had to get my old crock. The nursing supervisor was very careful not to reappear.

The nurses' heels on the floor tiles.

J.-F. M. told me, when I was in the other hospital, "if some day you have a problem that requires a few days of observation, they won't even find a bed for you because there aren't any. That's another reason why you have to change wards."

Read more than enough books in my life, wrote more than enough?

The day I learned that it was cytomegalovirus that had attacked my eye, alone in the outpatient room, I saw a huge black spider come out of a hole in the heating ducts.

Tonight, the heavily clouded sky lit by the moon is like a snowy field.

September 23

The right eye: I see three black butterflies pass across the light source.

They got me up at six forty-five to take my temperature. At seven, with the cup of coffee I got from the machine since the cafeteria was still closed, I enter the office near my room where all the nurses get together to drink their coffee and discuss the flow charts and organization of care. It's very bad for a patient to linger at the entrance to this room, I say: "I hope you will excuse me for troubling your conviviality but I will only be a second. Is the nurse who will administer my medication this morning one of you?" "Yes, me," answers a girl, after some hesitation. "You will have to find a hep-lock for me somewhere, either in the pharmacy or in another ward, because the last one was used yesterday evening." "What color is your needle?" "Pink." "I'll find one for you."

White roses (C.) and yellow roses (my sister) in my room.

T. and I can't even hug anymore, which was so comforting when we used to meet. It would be too melodramatic now.

I think that supplies must be stolen in hospitals, or else this wouldn't be possible. I wonder what it must be like in Russia!

Chirac's "smell," Cresson's "charters," Giscard's "invasion," independent of my state, I will never vote again in my life.

J.-F. M. has his own tube so he can be artificially fed from a machine, at the level of his heart.

Monday is better than Sunday, in the hospital and everywhere else.

My great-aunt Louise, who came yesterday to visit me
with my sister and her daughter, discovers television at the
age of eighty-five in her nursing home, and tells me of
outrageous peals of laughter while watching certain com-
edy shows.

Yesterday, it took me a long time to pick up the phone,
I finally recognize little Titou's tiny voice. We hadn't
seen each other since before the vacation. He seems very
moved. I am.

The morning nurse hid three hep-locks in my closet that
she took from cardiology.

It's difficult to have a sense of humor lying down: it seems
affected, given the lack of breath.

In the glass walkway that leads to the ward, street people.
They've taken their shoes because they were too filthy, and
given them blue paper slippers instead, and on their heads,
since they have lice, caps made from the same blue paper.
They look at me as I pass among them, head high, trying not to avoid them with my gaze as everyone is supposed to do.

Making mental torture (the situation in which I find
myself, for instance) a subject for study, even for a whole
work, makes the torture somewhat more bearable.

I gave the first notebook to H.G., in a sealed envelope, without telling him what it was, because tomorrow I'll go down to the operating room at nine o'clock and I was afraid they'd take it from me in my room, or even in my pocket.

Finally, a moving pole, it must have been stolen from someone, maybe. Someone died.

For the first time today, Monday, I listened to a little music on the radio (NJR, Radio Nostalgie, Radio Nova), programs prepared by T.

I found out from H.G., who heard it from B., who heard it from P., that V. called him to know where I was.

Dr. M., the anesthesiologist, who is supposed to install my port-a-cath tomorrow morning, came to see me this afternoon. He examined my torso and told me how it was supposed to go. I asked him a lot of questions, as usual. At a certain point, I told him, bare-chested, "I'm using you a little like a screen." My friend S. was sitting behind him, pretending to go through some mail. "She's very curious," I added.

There must be some nurses and orderlies who, at first sight and as a matter of principle, detest patients who have single rooms, since that means they're rich. Ninety francs a day.

I listen to old hits from my youth, which have no effect
on me.

I refused to let them give me a paper pillowcase today.

September 24

Whatever the operation, without thinking, they tell the
patient above all to fast, which isn't necessary two-thirds of
the time, but that way they won't get yelled at. The stomach
and psyche of the patient vanish in thin air.

The duty nurse told the petulant brunette nurse that I said,
"The type who still appeals to men." The nurse in question
repeats it to me while she's administering the IV, I'm ill
at ease, I try, at least, nonchalantly, to eliminate the word
"still" and repeat, "The type of woman who appeals to
men." She tells me kindly that, in any case, she took it well,
it flattered her, she says. I understand precisely why the
duty nurse repeated it: she herself is no longer pleasing to
men, not at all.

The bitch who made me enter the room that hadn't been
disinfected enters triumphantly at seven-thirty in the
morning with a transparent blue gown. She wants me to
strip and wear it, allowing me to keep my underwear. I tell
her: "You'll have to wait until I'm a lot worse off than I am
now to get me to walk through a hospital in this thing. The
only way you'll get me to accept would be to accompany

me, hand in hand, in the same outfit, and I'd authorize
you to keep your bra, just as you authorize me to keep my
underwear."

A young nurse would like to observe the operation, she's
never seen it before. I tell her, "You'd better wait until it's
a good looking, muscled hunk, with superb pecs, so then
you'd kill two birds with one stone."

Wrote nothing this evening. Too shell-shocked. I'll try
tomorrow.

September 25

Yesterday, a cursed day, bad luck, chain of catastrophes,
even though I wasn't in the least apprehensive about this
operation, I even had the premonition that it would go
very well.

The bitch's face when she saw me pass alone, in my street
clothes, my hat on my head, the transparent blue gown
over my shoulder, going toward the operating room: non-
plussed, there's no better word for it.

The only function of the transparent blue gown was
humiliation.

The expression on the faces of the orderlies, big Mada-
gascans dressed in light green from head to toe, when they

opened the door of the recovery room for me: "Who are
you? What are you doing?" I got undressed in the bathroom, and I too put on the green pajama bottoms without
any front or back, the green top, the green slippers, the
green cap.

Three hours in the operating room, instead of three-
quarters of an hour as planned. They went all out: twenty
deep punctures with big needles and burning xylocaine,
an artery entered a few millimeters from the aorta and
the jugular, the anesthesiologist sweating bullets, he said,
"We'll stop, I'm going for a cup of coffee, we can start
again later" (afterward I thought: Alcohol? Drugs?), they
take an ultrasound of the neck, they focus on a vein that
wouldn't be too thin and wouldn't roll, the needle enters
on the first try, it doesn't hurt, I can feel the incision in the
skin with the sharp blade that the anesthesiologist demanded from his assistants, hemorrhage, I tell them I feel
very poorly, I feel like I'm going to faint, oxygen mask that
has no effect, suddenly an intolerable pain near my heart, I
scream, I beg them to take away the pain, for a few seconds
I think I'm going to die; despite the hemorrhage they can't
stop, they have to sew me fast before the anesthesia wears
off. Morphine shot. They slide me from the operating table
to a cart, then to my bed. Recovery room. A big guy with
a bare chest whom they take away immediately, a young
Asian woman who seems asleep, and whose face shows the
signs of pain, a girl with big, open staring eyes, and, next
to me, a little hidden from view by the end of the bed, a

black man whose arm is saturated with IVs, he's very agitated, he's in pain, I understand that they've already given him the maximum dose of morphine. They tie him to the bed. I asked for a cup of coffee, delicious.

During the operation I suffocate under the paper covers that delineate the operation's parameters and prevent me from seeing what's going on. I'm in pain. I feel a tear roll from the corner of my right eyelid. Despite the difficulties we're going through, a nurse hums, a few seconds, that helps me.

I've been tortured for nothing: they didn't even try to drag the truth out of me.

I just saw a cadaver pass under a black shroud: recovery room.

When you enter the ICU, with its machines, noises, the annoying beep-beep, the open doors, the running in the hall, the nurses calling for help, you think at first that it's a new hell. Then I think it's the perfect place to die, they're needed.

I thought I would no longer be able to write in this diary because of the trauma, but it's the only way to forget.

When M. was in the ICU, a few weeks before he died, they had to put a guard in front of his door even though it was closed because they caught a photographer slipping into the room to take pictures of M., unconscious.

They all want to change jobs: get up at five-thirty, take public transportation at six, get off the bus and run to the hospital at seven to grab a cup of coffee with their sisters getting off the night shift.

The anesthesiologist who collapsed my lung yesterday came to chat with me yesterday evening and this morning. I just can't resist warming up to him.

Every day in the paper I check what the temperature is in Rome.

Comparing chest x-rays from yesterday and today. No chest tube for now. Total immobility.

Sometimes they just don't know anymore, they feel their way, they sweat buckets. They're afraid. They inject xylocaine between the pleura and the lung to be able to install the chest tube, a kind of small drain.

September 26

A nurse arrives, flustered, while they stick in the chest tube for the third time and she cries: "Mrs. X. is all marbled!" With her green nozzle, the nurse sprays the air, with a syringe, the air that they extract from my lungs. She says: "I feel like a fairy."

Jack hammer in the intensive care unit. Skimmed farmer's cheese, 5% fat for a patient who's lost twenty kilos.

Last evening, wait for the emergency ambulance unit: coma due to attempted suicide. The doctors in the ambulance unit are pissed off, the girl's family insulted them, called them delivery men. The girl groans, she swallowed pills and drank a lot of alcohol, she's in the room next to mine.

During the night, while I was sleeping very soundly, a nurse woke me up by just grazing my hand with one light finger.

I urinate without getting up, in a sort of condom tied to a tube, a Texas catheter. They put the freezing, sharp steel of the basin under my back, I can't do it. They give me a shot in the stomach with a short little needle to avoid scabs. Nothing bothers me anymore, except trepanning, and eye injections.

This morning, sad and discouraged. The kindness of the orderly who bathes me and puts me back to bed improves my morale a bit.

General strike in the hospital.

Curiously, at the moment of intense suffering exerted by
the doctor on the patient, a feeling of love and respect,
which I believe is reciprocal, is created. Suffering is somehow sacred. The doctor who caused the suffering and the
patient who suffered become friends in a way, accomplices,
but it's reserved.

The head critical care doctor came by with his assistant
and pulled out the tube stuck in my chest with a quick tug,
it was tied to a glass container filled with a purple liquid,
where my exhaling and my coughing should have made
bubbles. No bandage, so five minutes later, a small, dry red
dot on my chest, much smaller than the tube that was in
there. The mysteries of the body.

September 27

Left the ICU yesterday evening to go back to the regular
ward, room 366. I got a lot of rest. Severe case of candidia-
sis in the throat. Bright sunshine.

This morning, while trying to shave, I saw in the mirror
an abnormally enlarged artery above the port-a-cath, which
was a little painful.

Two nurses came to clean me up. I told them I would do it
myself. I haven't gotten up for two days. They were afraid
I'd fall in the bathroom.

It wasn't an artery, but rather a tube beneath the skin.

The psychiatrist came to see me yesterday evening, not very thrilled because I never came back to see him in his office, though it is near my apartment. He writes in my file: "To-day, the patient is calm. Thoughtful discourse." The last time, discourse was "coherent."

I can picture myself in a white neck brace, a black patch over one eye if it's done for, with a great hat. In that case, I would again agree to be photographed.

This morning, when they came to get me with a wheelchair to take me to radiology (with its drafts, it's the sort of environment that inflicts pulmonary problems on those who are free of them), I first hid my notebook under the pillow and then I told myself that was a very bad idea; since it fit I put it in my shirt pocket.

This evening, I ate the raspberries H.G. brought. It's one of the last things my great-aunt Suzanne liked to eat when she was ninety-five years old.

Today, I proudly celebrated my sister's birthday, but it was yesterday.

When I was hospitalized at the Rothschild, that hospital was also on strike. When I was hospitalized at the Spallan-zani in Rome, the nurses there were also on strike.

September 28

There are nurses who love their job. I got to know one in
the intensive care unit, very young, pretty, precise, coura-
geous. There is nothing more terrific for a patient. Only
in the evening, when she leaves the hospital at 10 P.M. to go
home, she's worn out.

I asked C. to get me coffee from the machine on the
ground floor, 100% Arabica, sugar, hit the "robust" but-
ton. But she goes up the hall and brings me back a little
espresso from the cafeteria, which is of better quality. Only
there's a lot less liquid to burn my throat, the way I like it,
but I never mention it to her.

The woman responsible for experimental therapies invited
me to dinner with her family in her house in Chagny. She
says she would have driven me back to the hospital.

The Madagascan cleaning woman and I have been talking
to each other on a first name basis since the first day, and
we both enjoy it.

Cough during the night. Cavernous noise in the pneumothorax. Bad sleep.

T., my good friend, only comes to see me once a week, on
Saturday afternoons. He has his work, his kids, the long
ride to the hospital. Nothing gives me more pleasure than

this visit and yet it's so melancholy each time that I dread it as much as I look forward to it: between us, we have our youth—which is lost—and our eroticism—which is also lost—that brings us together. What remains is a great love, greater than ever.

I force myself to eat. Long live yogurts, puddings, sweets!

Tomorrow, change from summer to winter time.

September 29

Sunday morning. I sunbathe in the Paris suburbs, behind double glass windows.

Little Titou, who never showed me much affection, except when I brought him gifts, obstinately asks to see me, he must have a premonition.

Sundays, there are croissants.

A tune on the hit parade: *Le dormeur doit se réveiller* (*The Sleeper Must Awaken*).

Yesterday evening, the nurse who came for my IV tried first to inject a normal saline solution to clear the port-a-cath. It doesn't work, no matter how much she tries to push the syringe, it doesn't go through. "It's blocked," she says. "And so what do you do when it's blocked?" "We change the syringe, in case that's the problem." "Are you sure you made all the connections?" "Ah, good thing you mentioned that, I forgot to check." The heart beats again.

This morning, a kind intern came to announce that my pneumothorax must not have been resorbed, since the x-ray showed a big pocket of air under my collapsed lung. When they first read the x-ray, they told me it had been completely resorbed, a few days later, uneasily, they told me there was a little bubble of air that would disappear by itself. I take some syrup. I hurt a little. I'm very pessimistic about what's to come.

This morning, the head of the clinic came to offer me permission to leave until 8 P.M., because of the beautiful weather. Take a stroll on the highway?

All you hear here is: "Have a good meal!" "Have a good day!" "Have a good weekend!" "Have a good night!" "Have a good vacation!" never "Have a good death."

After my doctor, who thought it was meningitis, told me for the first time with authority, "If we don't find any-thing on the scan, Mr. Guibert, I absolutely want to do a lumbar puncture," his assistant grabbed me in the hall and whispered: "Don't let them do the lumbar puncture, Mr. Guibert." A few days later, after the complications with the port-a-cath, she tells me: "You didn't see the face I was making when they talked about the port-a-cath?"

V. told me he would stop by this Sunday. He didn't come, and didn't even call. I thought this was so shitty of him that I didn't dare admit it to my other friends.

The people in the rooms down the hall, mostly in pajamas and in pairs, do everything to pass the time: TV, radio, parlor games, electronic games, smoking in the glass walkway. Me, I don't do anything to pass the time. I nap.

Some orderlies have a strategy: they make such a face when you buzz for the smallest necessary service that you would rather swim in your own diarrhea than see those ugly mugs, tired, debilitating, almost nasty sometimes.

September 30

Isn't it cruel to have given no news to my parents after giving them the news that I was going to be hospitalized for two weeks, without elaborating—or else my mother would have bombarded my answering machine with tearful, supplicating messages—and to have forbidden them moreover from seeking details through intermediaries like T. and C., or my sister? But wouldn't the cruelty I would inflict on myself by calling them be even more cruel? Furthermore, what would I say to them? "Everything's fine," or else "I may become blind, they gave me a pneumothorax and collapsed a lung during an operation, I had a hemorrhage, I stayed completely immobile in the ICU for two days, I'm in despair and I have no desire to see you." They always

claim that they would want to suffer in my place, because
that isn't possible.

The orderly, frizzy-haired and bold, when she came yesterday morning to make my bed and to change my sheets even
though it's a weekend—"You must have sweated quite a
bit last night, Mr. Guibert, or am I wrong?"—describes in
detail (including the itineraries) all the beautiful trips she
took with her ex-husband: Italy, Spain, Portugal—"we just
passed through." She lived in Dunkerque, so on Saturday
nights she would cross the border into Belgium to go danc-
ing: "They know how to have a good time up North. . . ."
What she really loves is to travel. She's getting ready to go
to Oklahoma.

The hospital is freezing, everyone is coughing.

The ophthalmologist told me this morning that, contrary
to what they had told me, they often collapse a lung while
installing a port-a-cath. I asked her if the nodules rested
on the optic nerve, she told me: "No, on the cornea." The
fundus of the eye under dilation does not register light
through the cornea, now that I'm almost no longer afraid
of it. Apparently no improvement, she wants ten more days
of aggressive treatment. I give her my book *Des aveugles*, with
the dedication "Explanation of an obsession?" I asked her
if blindness provoked by the CMV is partial or total [*une
cécité blanche, ou noire*]. She answers, "It changes as the virus ad-
vances." She's going to prescribe glasses for me so I can read.

There is nothing left here: no spoon, no sugar, no bowl, no pillowcase, no heat, no paper towels, no tissue paper, it's Russia, or the Villa Medici.

October 1

This morning, a man's little wispy voice, not at all aggressive, asks the Madagascan cleaning woman to go through the garbage can she's emptying to look for a little notebook that he must have thrown away by accident or his roommate—though he doesn't want to accuse anyone—might have thrown away out of nastiness. But the Madagascan cleaning woman doesn't want to hear about it: "A garbage can is a garbage can," she says, "what's in there doesn't come out again." "You must understand," says the little wispy voice with even greater modesty, "it was full of notes that I jotted down, which couldn't really interest anyone in the world but me."

Morale was improving slowly, like a snail at the bottom of a mountain. And then the social worker came to tell me that I won't get out Thursday, but next Tuesday.

October 2

One more day to get through. A day of near-despair. The only thing that gives me some pleasure is to go back to my soft bed.

Last wishes: incinerated, as soon as possible. No religious ceremony, no gathering of friends and family at the moment of cremation, no music. Throw away the ashes in the first garbage can.

October 3

Morale a bit improved today. H., who came to visit this morning, very smartly dressed, white shirt, polka dot tie, three-piece suit and raincoat, black briefcase, rushing by before his first appointment, thinks that the Prozac must be starting to have some effect, he says it takes between ten to twenty days, we calculated it's been thirteen since I took the first pill. If only it could continue to do me some good. I've been so low these last few days.

Yesterday morning, in the hall leading to radiology, sitting naked on a cart, the bottom half of his body hidden by a sheet, a young man covered in dried blood. A white bandage at the level of his spinal column. They must have given him a spinal tap. He doesn't want to lie down, he resists, his arms locked behind his body to hold himself up. Everything in that body is sublime: its power, its elegance, the joint linking the arm to the shoulder. . . . When I rediscover an erotic emotion, it's like finding a bit of life while drowning in this sea of death [*bain de mort*].

The other morning, the orderly who came to take me to ophthalmology on a stretcher even though I didn't need his help since I could walk by myself was very irritated by my blue hat; he wanted me to take it off and said: "You don't need that to go to ophthalmology." I tell him, "What did my hat ever do to you?" He sulks a little. I'm able to calm him down by giving him a false clue to the riddle "My head's freezing."

"What can you possibly do with all the thermometers that they leave for you here?" the gorgeous, vigorous hunk with the little diamond stud in his ear asks me. "I eat them." He says, "So mercury's your thing, huh?"

When I close my left eye to see out of my right eye, the object observed is erased slowly from the bottom up, until it becomes invisible, nonexistent.

A little bit in love with the thermometer man. It's enjoyable. He's cheerful.

October 4

With Z., who came to see me the other day bringing a stuffed animal, a boxing monkey with a tender yet menacing expression, we talk about burial and incineration. She buried her mother, who wanted to be incinerated but hadn't left any written record of her wishes. She thinks we should respect the tradition of waiting three days to give the dead the chance to leave. You light a candle behind their head. You don't wash them, you don't put make-up on them, you leave them in the clothes they had on when they died. No heat, of course, but no draft either. For the burial, friends accompany the dead to the tomb, where they throw cut flowers, then they get together in a café to talk warmly about the dead person. This is quite a ways from ashes thrown into the first available garbage can.

The afternoon wears on. I can't wait for the night to come, forgetting.

Silence, eyes closed. Unbearable radio.

I didn't bring my camera.

October 5

Fog. Besides the neon sign above a garage entrance, you can't see a thing. The sun came up and is glaring off the window. But tonight, the orderlies say, it'll be quite cold.

October 6

Nothing. It's Sunday. The hospital has finally won?

Tried to reread a little, without too much difficulty (*Promenades* by Carl Seelig, with Robert Walser), what a joy!

So frustrated from lack of reading that I really push it, I force it, I devour.

October 7

I read, sitting in the sun in the armchair, waiting for my IV
to drain.

Slept poorly. Nightmares about the port-a-cath, with all
its tubes and connections, that scared T. yesterday when he
asked me to show him. I only found out last night that I
will not be able to bathe or shower more than once a week
when the needle comes out.

This morning in radiology I tripped getting up from the
chair and fell on my knees. An old man, who looked a bit
like a gypsy, told me I should eat more.

October 8

I read (only today, by chance) that DHPG, the antiviral
that they perfuse into me every day, irreversibly blocks the
production of sperm, but I don't give a fuck about fucking
right now.

The noise of a squeaking cart sounds like the songs of
birds.

Among the undesirable side effects listed on the insert in
the medication package: "abnormal dreams." Dreams a few
days apart of two nude women lying on my gaunt body.

I leave the hospital. HHC = home health care. Absolute horror: "rehos" (nurse's abbreviation for "rehospitalization").

Writing in the dark?

Writing until the end?

Putting an end to it so as not to end up fearing death?

Remainders

TODD MEYERS

But of all this daily drama of the body there is no record.

—Virginia Woolf, *On Being Ill* (1930)

Thirty years have passed since Robert Gallo identified the retrovirus associated with AIDS, while at the same time in France, Luc Montagnier and colleagues at the Institut Pasteur isolated a "lymphadenopathy-associated virus" (LAV), the virus now called HIV.[1] This moment of mutual discovery, heralded and eternized, was not a turning point but occurred along a continuum of uncertainty, controversy, legacy, anger, and loss—and in our present moment, such loss has evolved to include overwriting (historical, fantastical) and distancing (geographical, generational).

The year of Hervé Guibert's death is the year the U.S. Department of Health and Human Services proposes to remove HIV from the list of diseases used to bar entry into the United States. It is the same year a famous American basketball player announces he is HIV positive.[2] It is the first year funds from the Ryan White Comprehensive AIDS Resources Emergency Act are allocated. And while it is important not to mistake a French story for an Anglo-American one, it is difficult to ignore the rhyming between sites of the epidemic, even if there remain different scales and momentums globally.[3] Still, Guibert's book arrives at a moment of special importance in the history of AIDS—a history very much in and of the present—and finds its way into the space between facets of the epidemic, in two distinct national contexts.[4] The book is of presence and actuality, of living and the animation of thought, at a time when the philosophical stakes of *being* were under threat.[5] And yet questions of citizenship, belonging, political action, and public withdrawal reside in the background of Guibert's hospitalization diary. In a moment remembered for its public health crises and grand political gestures—which tend to overshadow the smaller battles of an already embattled health care system, with its strained resources, staffing crises, misunderstanding and fear across many publics[6]—Guibert offers a spectacularly slight account.

Guibert is hospitalized as AZT and promising new ddI and ddC drugs become increasingly available thanks to pressure from gay and lesbian activists. The "compassionate" access to experimental therapies is regularized only months after Guibert's death. It was the unregulated sharing of trial drugs that Guibert had taken out of the shadow of mutual aid, failure, and concealment, placing the intimacies formed in and through these therapies in full light.[7] While antiretroviral therapies were the focus, activists were also at odds with the producers and regulators of treatment drugs for cytomegalovirus retinitis.[8] Cytomegalovirus retinitis was the most serious ocular complication of AIDS, related most commonly to the reactivation of latent infection.[9] It is cytomegalovirus, or rather the threat of blindness, that is bound up with a sense of a life's being eclipsed in Guibert's writing. As Guibert suggests, *Cytomegalovirus* is a backward premonition, an anticipation of blindness, of death, and of other forms of loss, as a kind of flattening of the self or what makes the individual.[10]

Cytomegalovirus straddles or bends the genres of philosophy and literature—and, now, years into the AIDS epidemic, history. The writing is filled with humor, an avoidance of sentimentality, pedestrian moments of complaining about hospital food, poor sheets, petty battles with nurses, boredom, all rendered sparsely and forcefully in a way that retains a double character unique to Guibert's circumstance while moving outside of it. Echoes of *Cytomegalovirus* can be heard, accidentally and unmistakably, in the most familiar moments of Jean-Luc Nancy's philosophy, especially his *L'Intrus*.[11] Nancy's attempt to disentangle "the organic, the symbolic, the imaginary," in his case of a heart transplant, shares with *Cytomegalovirus* the strange and uncanny "sensation of falling overboard while remaining on deck."[12] Even the mode of writing finds kinship ("To defer death is to also exhibit it, to underscore it."[13]). There is a distinction that is collapsed between what is foreign and the self (for Nancy the intruder that is simultaneously "I," for Thomas Mann the sickening of matter and reception of the primordial, for Virginia Woolf to become a deserter in the army of the upright), making Guibert something other than a correspondent from the epidemic.[14]

Cytomegalovirus is blunt and unrehearsed. Guibert tells us that his hospital diary helps to give "rhythm to time and a way to pass it"; he also gives for his reader a rhythm to thought and draws us into his corporal orbit: the darkness and light and imbalance of his hospital room, as it shrinks, oceans between the bathroom and the bed widen, the celestial mooring to the IV pole tightens, the sky seen through the frame of the window charts distance and scale. Guibert calls our attention to the objects that surround him, as he turns along their revolution. Like the photographs of Nan Goldin, who at the same time was making images of her dying friends, Guibert struggles to produce "the real of this real," emptied by an unseen hand, its probing intrusion, its qualities of exposure and suffering.[15] Guibert's is a galaxy of refusals, resignations, muted wit, vulnerability—but none familiar with his voice will find him estranged from it. There is feltness and withdrawal against the expected prose of despair. Jean-Pierre Boulé writes that there are two main characters in *Cytomegalovirus*: Guibert and death.[16] But there is a third, a remainder, something we could even call the remainder of living as a subject shaped beyond Guibert, no matter how spare or twisted (for once he is twisted, not the twister). Clara Orban suggests that Guibert is writing *toward* the dying body as the way of "writing to the end," which I take to mean "at," as the end *receives* writing, and "until," as a time signature.[17] If there is discomfort with its genre, then it is because *Cytomegalovirus* does not fit easily as *memoir* or *pathography* or *thanatographical writing* but establishes itself as *life writing*, or writing on the side of life, in its strictest sense.

Cytomegalovirus blends the public and private, anticipates a public, but in a mode very different from his actual journals, recently translated into English as *The Mausoleum of Lovers*.[18] Here we find a distinctive need, not exposé;[19] secrets are not so much revealed as discovered.[20] Whereas *The Mausoleum of Lovers* may be sensual, obscene, without determination but with a healthy self-awareness from the outset, here Guibert follows Woolf's "childish outspokenness in illness" wherein "things are said, truths blurted out,"[21] which are just as readily concealed or realized carefully in light of what can be recorded in a physically diminished state, "at" or "until" the end.

Hervé Guibert's *Cytomegalovirus* is singular—banal, beautiful, truthful. Yet the book contravenes the notion of a narrative that holds *a* bare truth; Guibert happily muddles the valorized voice of the patient and calls into question valor itself. Another writer, whose relation to pain and death found equally sharp and uneasy prose, in his case during the time of Proust's Paris, is Alphonse Daudet. In the introduction to Daudet's *In the Land of Pain*, Julian Barnes remarks, "[W]hat happens around illness may be dramatic, even heroic; but illness is ordinary; day-to-day, boring."[22] Daudet shows through the shudder of tertiary syphilis that pain is always new to the sufferer, losing originality only for those around him.[23] It is a continual phenomenon in everyday life with an expression that belies this fact.[24] Daudet is fierce when he states that there is "no general theory about pain. Each patient discovers his own, and the nature of pain varies, like a singer's voice, according to the acoustics of the hall."[25] For Guibert, the hospital room, the touch of his words to the sheets and the walls, the objects and the body, find their unique register.

In what sense is this a philosophy of life or of living? The appearance of the book in a series entitled "Forms of Living" requires some explanation, or perhaps punctuation. First is the question of its philosophical stakes, which in part are found in the philosophical anthropology of Michel Foucault—an effort to make visible that which is already visible.[26] In Guibert's hospitalization diary we are confronted with a scene of life at its eclipse, where the terms of that life are in the midst of their founding. Yet *Cytomegalovirus* does not feed on its own concepts—it is not a comment on life; it is an expression of what Georges Canguilhem marks as the arrival of new norms in and of the body, for *an individual.*[27] There is no generalization, no concepts cleaving for expression. *Cytomegalovirus* is not "medical subjectivism" but rather a work at "that margin of tolerance" of health, where such things are made real—ordinary concepts no longer hold sway, the simplicity of prose overwhelms, and catastrophe is sensed. As Virginia Woolf writes:

> All day, all night the body intervenes ... unending change, heat and cold, comfort and discomfort, hunger and satisfaction, health and illness, until there comes the

inevitable catastrophe; the body smashes itself to smith-
ereens, and the soul (it is said) escapes. But of all this
daily drama of the body there is no record.[28]

But here we find a record, a remainder, of this daily drama.

NOTES

1. Steven Epstein, *Impure Science: AIDS, Activism, and the Politics of
Knowledge*. Berkeley: University of California Press, 1996.
2. G. A. Gellert et al., "Disclosure of AIDS in Celebrities." *New
England Journal of Medicine* 1992; 327: 1389.
3. See David Caron, *AIDS in French Culture*. Madison: University of
Wisconsin Press, 2001; Epstein, *Impure Science*; Victoria Harden, *AIDS
at 30: A History*. Dulles, Va.: Potomac Books, 2012.
4. Hervé Guibert's *Cytomégalovirus: Journal d'hospitalisation* was published in 1992, and the original English edition in 1996.
5. Paula A. Treichler, *How to Have Theory in an Epidemic: Cultural
Chronicles of AIDS*. Durham, N.C.: Duke University Press, 1999; see also
Emily Apter's important essay "Fantom Images: Hervé Guibert and
the Writing of 'Sida' in France," in *Writing AIDS: Gay Literature, Language,
and Analysis*, ed. Timothy F. Murphy and Suzanne Poirier. New York:
Columbia University Press, 1993, 83–97.
6. Ronald Bayer, *Private Acts, Social Consequences: AIDS and the Politics
of Public Health*. New York: Free Press, 1989; National Academy of
Sciences, *Confronting AIDS: Update 1988*. Washington: National Academy Press 1988, 108.
7. Hervé Guibert, *The Compassion Protocol*, trans. James Kirkup. New
York: Braziller, 1994.
8. A. G. Palestine et al. "A randomized, controlled trial of fos-
carnet in the treatment of cytomegalovirus retinitis in patients with
AIDS." *Annals of Internal Medicine* 1991; 115(9): 665–73.
9. W. Byne, "Cytomegalovirus," *GMHC Treatment Issues Compilation*.
New York: Gay Men's Health Crisis, Nov. 1987–March 1989, 57.

10. His earlier novel, *Des aveugles* (Of the blind, translated as *Blindsight*) Paris: Gallimard, 1985, deals with the topic of blindness; see also Ralph Sarkonak, *Angelic Echoes: Hervé Guibert and Company*. Toronto: University of Toronto Press, 2000, 170.

11. Jean-Luc Nancy, *L'Intrus*. Paris: Galilée, 2000.

12. Ibid., 15: ". . . de passer par-dessus bord en restant sur le pont."

13. Ibid., 25: "Différer la mort, c'est aussi l'exhiber, la souligner."

14. Sarkonak, *Angelic Echoes*, 204.

15. See Michael Bracewell, "Making Up Is Hard to Do." *Frieze* 1993, Issue 12, on the photographs of Nan Goldin; Hervé Guibert, *Ghost Image*, trans. Robert Bononno. Chicago: University of Chicago Press, 2014.

16. Jean-Pierre Boulé, *Hervé Guibert: Voices of the Self*, trans. John Fletcher. Liverpool: Liverpool University Press, 1999, 232.

17. Clara Orban, *Body [in] Parts: Bodies and Identity in Sade and Guibert*. Lehigh, Pa.: Lehigh University Press, 2008, 18, 37.

18. Hervé Guibert, *The Mausoleum of Lovers: Journals 1976–1991*, trans. Nathanaël. New York: Nightboat, 2014.

19. Hervé Guibert, *Mes parents*. Paris: Gallimard, 1986.

20. See Sarkonak, *Angelic Echoes.*

21. Virginia Woolf, *On Being Ill*. New York: Paris Press, 2002, 11.

22. Julian Barnes, "Introduction" to Alphonse Daudet, *In the Land of Pain*, trans. Julian Barnes. New York: Knopf, 2002, xiii–xvi.

23. Daudet, *In the Land of Pain*, 19.

24. Joanna Bourke, *The Story of Pain*. Oxford: Oxford University Press, 2014, 228; see René Leriche, *La chirurgie de la douleur*. Paris: Masson & Cie, 1940.

25. Daudet, *In the Land of Pain*, 15.

26. Michel Foucault, *Dits et écrits, tome 1: 1954–1975*. Paris: Gallimard, 1978, 540–41.

27. Georges Canguilhem, *Writings on Medicine*, trans. Stefanos Geroulanos and Todd Meyers. New York: Fordham University Press, 2012; see also Stefanos Geroulanos and Todd Meyers, *Experimente im individuum, Kurt Goldstein und die Frage des Organismus*, trans. Nils F. Schott and Holger Wölfle. Berlin: August Verlag, 2013.

28. Woolf, *On Being Ill*, 4–5.

Cytomegalovirus is a slight work whose style is elliptical and dense at times, at others lyrical and colloquial. The text presents Guibert's intimate observations during a three-week hospital stay while he confronts his fears about end-stage AIDS and the cytomegalovirus threatening him with blindness. He remains a keen observer of the world of the hospital ward, recording the most intimate details of his life as a patient in his diary. He depicts the people he meets— doctors, patients, friends who come to visit—and the effect they have on him. He also describes with great clarity the sometimes degrading role the patient plays in the hospital drama. Throughout, he defiantly clings to his human dignity, refusing to be treated like an object of study or of compassion. He demands to be a part of every procedure the hospital staff performs on him so that until the end, his body will remain his own.

Most important, writing is a way of recording his experience and therefore of preserving his humanity. Writing is crucial to survival for Guibert, and impending blindness threatens this lifeline. Like an IV, the notebook he hides in his hospital room represents a link to life, to conquering the AIDS virus that ravages him. The final words of the text are posed as a question, when Guibert poignantly wonders whether he will "write until the end."

I was introduced to Guibert's work more than twenty years ago. For a Comparative Literature seminar on Images of Disease in Twentieth Century Literature in autumn 1994, I translated this work to share with students at DePaul University. A colleague, Pascale-Anne Brault, had introduced me to the power and beauty of Guibert's prose and photographs. Several of his other works had already been translated into English, but this one seemed most appropriate for the group of undergraduates that quarter. She and another colleague, Andrew Suozzo, knew Guibert's work well and offered guidance as I chose my class materials.

I subsequently published the first English-language translation of this text in 1996. Pascale-Anne Brault and Michael Naas were very generous with their time, and I found their expert advice on the translation draft invaluable.

In 2014, Todd Meyers approached me about reissuing the translation in a format more accessible to students and general readers. He believes in this text and has found it useful as a teaching tool, as I had so many years before. I am forever grateful to him and to his co-editor, Stefanos Geroulanos, in the "Forms of Living" series with Fordham University Press for making the current reissue a reality. Fordham University

Press and its board have been wonderful to work with as we moved forward.

Most of all, however, my husband, Elliot Weisenberg, M.D., was unfailing in his assistance with this project. As I confronted medical or hospital terminology that was unfamiliar, he helped find the right words to bring the French text to an English audience. *Cytomegalovirus* is similar to a poem—compact, where every word resonates more fully because of the brevity of the text. Each word that he helped bring to life makes this text richer.

Clara Orban

DePaul University, Chicago

November 2014

Printed and bound by CPI Group (UK) Ltd, Croydon, CR0 4YY

27/10/2024

14580328-0001